MW01232351

Sirtfood Diet for Beginners

The complete guide with easy, tasty and healthy recipes to lose weight, burn fat and feel good with Sirtfood

The information in the following pages is broadly considered a truthful and accurate account of facts and as such, any inattention, use, or misuse of the information in question by the reader will render any resulting actions solely under their purview. There are no scenarios in which the publisher or the original author of this work can be in any fashion deemed liable for any hardship or damages that may befall them after undertaking information described herein.

Additionally, the information in the following pages is intended only for informational purposes and should thus be thought of as universal. As befitting its nature, it is presented without assurance regarding its prolonged validity or interim quality. Trademarks that are mentioned are done without written consent and can in no way be considered an endorsement from the trademark holder.

TABLE OF CONTENTS

BREAKFAST

White Beans with Lemon

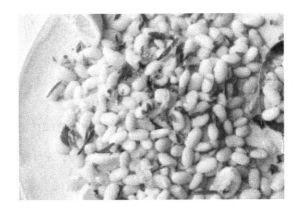

Preparation time: 5 minutes

Cooking time: 10 minutes

Servings: 1

Ingredients:

- A jar of white beans from Spain
- Breadcrumbs
- 4 Lemons
- A teaspoon of extra virgin olive oil
- A big onion

Directions:

1. Cut the onion into fillets, put them in a pan with a little water and oil and cook. After a few minutes add the beans (rinse well under the tap). Stir and let it cook for a few minutes. Add salt, oil and breadcrumbs and mix. After a while, pour the lemon juice. Wait a little longer... and the dish is ready. Add more lemon at the end of cooking and eat!

Nutrition: Calories: 314 Net carbs: 51.6g Fat: 2.5g Fiber: 9.9g Protein: 14.1g

Sponge Beans with Onion

Preparation time: 10 minutes

Cooking time: 3 hours

Servings: 2

Ingredients:

- 250 g boiled Spanish beans
- 1 red onion
- 1 parsley
- Salt
- 2 teaspoons oil
- 1 teaspoon apple vinegar
- 1 teaspoon dried oregano or 5 fresh oregano leaves

Directions:

1. Cut the onion into thin slices and cook it for a minute with water in the microwave at full power. Combine all the ingredients in a bowl and leave to rest a couple of hours before serving, stirring a couple of times so that the beans take on the flavor of the seasoning.

Nutrition: Calories: 832 Net carbs: 23.1g Fat: 11.1g
Fiber: 13.9g Protein: 38.1g

Chickling Falafel

Preparation time: 24 hours

Cooking time: 30 minutes

Servings: 2

Ingredients:

- Half onion
- 200 grams chickling peas already soaked
- 80g of chickpea flour
- A teaspoon of cumin seed
- A clove of garlic
- Paprika

Directions:

1. Blend the chickling peas (previously soaked for 24 hours) together with the chopped onion, cumin, paprika, and garlic and chickpea flour. Blend until a fairly homogeneous mixture is obtained. Compact in a bowl and leave to rest in the fridge for about an hour. Take the dough and form some meatballs that will be baked in the oven at 180 degrees until golden brown. Notes Cumin can be reduced or eliminated completely.

Nutrition: Calories: 57 Net carbs: 5.4g Fat: 3g Protein: 2.2g

Chickpeas and Potato Omelette

Preparation time: 10 minutes

Cooking time: 25 minutes

Servings: 2

Ingredients:

- 4 teaspoons full of chickpea flour
- Olive oil
- Small potatoes

Directions:

1. This dish is very similar to the traditional 'omelette', but it is better and less heavy. It can be made with any vegetable, as well as potatoes (zucchini, spinach, onion, carrots, etc.). Put the chickpea flour in a soup plate, add 2 pinches of salt, and a little at a time water, stirring with a fork, until the dough is not too thick. Cut the potatoes into very thin slices, with the special blade of the grater or potato peeler, and pour them into the batter, stirring well. Put a little olive oil in a non-stick frying pan and heat over high heat. When the oil is hot, pour the mixture,

quickly distribute it evenly and put the lid on, leaving the heat high. Both the lid and the lively fire are important to get an omelette cooked to perfection! After about a minute, you have to turn the omelette: you can do it, if you are not able to turn it all over, by cutting it with a wooden shovel, in four slices, and turning one slice at a time. Put the lid back on for one more minute, leaving the fire lower. Then remove the lid, turn the omelette again and cook over high heat for one minute without lid, then turn again and cook for another minute, or until the omelette is golden on both sides.

Nutrition: Calories: 198 Net carbs: Fat: 4.4g Fiber: 8.4g Protein: 5.3g

Chickpea and Seed Omelette

Preparation time: 10 minutes

Cooking time: 25 minutes

Servings: 4

Ingredients:

- 5 teaspoons chickpea flour
- 1 teaspoon salt
- Olive oil 1 teaspoon
- Sesame seeds 1 teaspoon
- Linseed

Directions:

1. Pour the chickpea flour into a bowl, half a glass of water and mix well with force to remove any lumps of flour. Continue stirring, adding salt and sesame and linseed, for a few minutes until a thick cream is obtained. Heat the olive oil in the non-stick pan and pour the mixture over low heat. Prick the edges and the middle part with the fork and check that the bottom part does not stick to the bottom. It must not have a golden color,

so turn it as soon as the cream is absorbed and cook a few more minutes.

Nutrition: Calories: 209 Net carbs: 36.3g Fat: 0.9g Fiber: 8.9g Protein: 5.6g

Gluten Omelette

Preparation time: 1 hour 25 minutes

Cooking time: 6 minutes

Servings: 2

Ingredients:

- 1 kg of flour
- Olive oil
- 2 pinches of vegetable cube
- A handful of parsley
- A few drops of lemon
- Half a of salt

Directions:

1. First we have to get the gluten, and then we put the flour in a container and knead it with water as if we wanted to make bread. Let the dough rest for about an hour. After the resting period, we take our loaf of bread, tear off a piece not too big and wash it under water until only the gluten remains in our hands (the rinse water must remain almost transparent, no longer white as at

the beginning); we repeat the operation for the rest of the pasta.

2. Having finally obtained our gluten, iron it with our hands until it forms a medallion about one cm thick, put it in a pot, cover it with water (not too much, just enough to cover it), add half a of salt and boil it for 6 minutes, being careful not to stick it on the bottom and turn it on the other side halfway through cooking. We take our gluten out of the water and squeeze it with a fork to make it lose the excess liquid, pour the olive oil into a large pan and fry the gluten. While frying, we put a pinch of dice on both sides, chopped parsley and a few drops of lemon. As soon as it's golden and crisp it'll be ready. Place it on blotting paper and serve with a few drops of lemon and a nice salad.

Nutrition: Calories: 381 Net carbs: 4.6g Fat: 11.8g Fiber: 0.5g Protein: 34.4g

Tomato and Mushroom Omelette

Preparation time: 10 minutes

Cooking time: 15 minutes

Servings: 2

Ingredients:

- 4 teaspoons of chickpea flour
- 5 medium tomatoes
- One medium onion one
- Can of mushrooms
- Baking powder one
- Glass of water
- 1/4 of lemon oil for frying to taste

Directions:

1. Thinly slice the onion and fry it for 5 minutes, then add the chopped tomatoes and drained mushrooms; let it run on medium heat until the water that the tomatoes will tend to release has dried. In a plate, mix the chickpea flour with baking powder, a pinch of salt, a splash of lemon and a glass of water. Make sure the mixture is as velvety as possible and pour it into the pan. Fry

for 5 minutes stirring continuously. Dust with a spoonful of yeast and serve.

Nutrition: Calories: 173 Net carbs: 5.8g Fat: 3.2g Fiber: 1g Protein: 8g

Soy and Zucchini Omelette

Preparation time: 10 minutes

Cooking time: 10 minutes

Servings: 2

Ingredients:

- 2 small zucchini (100 g)
- 3 teaspoons of flour 00 (40 g)
- 2 pinches of salt
- 1/3 third glass of soy milk (60 g)
- 2 teaspoons of olive oil

Directions:

1. Cut the zucchini into very thin slices (with a greater with the appropriate blade, or with a potato peeler, not with a knife). Put the flour and salt in a soup plate, add the soy milk a little at a time and 2 fingers of water, and stir quickly with a fork so as not to form lumps. You have to get a batter that's not too dense, quite liquid. Pour in the zucchini slices and stir well. In a non-stick frying pan put 2 s of oil (so as to cover the bottom just barely) and heat over a high heat. When the

oil is hot, pour the batter and level well with a wooden spatula. Put the lid on it and leave the fire high, then after about half a minute lower the fire a little. The omelette must cook in all about 10 minutes, and in this time should be turned a couple of times, so that both sides are browned (you can cut it into 4 slices and turn them one at a time). Hold the lid for the first 5 minutes, for the remaining 5 minutes let it brown without the lid.

Nutrition: Calories: 115 Net carbs: 24.4g Fat: 0.6g Fiber: 4.6g Protein: 5.6g

Turkey Satay Skewers

Preparation time: 10 minutes

Cooking time: 10 minutes

Servings: 2

Ingredients:

- 250g turkey breast, cubed
- 25g smooth peanut butter
- 1 clove of garlic, crushed
- ½ small bird's eye chili (or more if you like it hotter), finely chopped
- ½ teaspoon ground turmeric
- 200mls coconut milk
- 2 teaspoons soy sauce

Directions:

1. Combine the coconut milk, peanut butter, turmeric, soy sauce, garlic and chili. Add the turkey pieces to the bowl and stir them until they are completely coated. Push the turkey onto metal skewers. Place the satay skewers on a barbeque or under a hot grill (broiler) and cook

for 4-5 minutes on each side, until they are completely cooked.

Nutrition: Calories: 431 Fat: 0.9g Protein: 4g

Salmon and Capers

Preparation time: 10 minutes

Cooking time: 5 minutes

Servings: 4

Ingredients:

- 75g Greek yogurt
- 4 salmon fillets, skin removed
- 4 teaspoons Dijon Mustard
- 1 capers, chopped
- 2 teaspoons fresh parsley
- Zest of 1 lemon

Directions:

1. In a bowl, mix together the yogurt, mustard, lemon zest, parsley and capers. Thoroughly coat the salmon in the mixture. Place the salmon under a hot grill (broiler) and cook for 3-4 minutes on each side, or until the fish is cooked. Serve with mashed potatoes and vegetables or a large green leafy salad.

Nutrition: Calories: 321 Fat: 6.7g Protein: 24.5g

Moroccan Chicken Casserole

Preparation time: 20 minutes

Cooking time: 50 minutes

Servings: 4

Ingredients:

- 250g tinned chickpeas (garbanzo beans) drained
- 4 chicken breasts, cubed
- 4 medjool dates, halved
- 6 dried apricots, halved
- 1 red onion, sliced
- 1 carrot, chopped
- 1 teaspoon ground cumin
- 1 teaspoon ground cinnamon
- 1 teaspoon ground turmeric
- 1 bird's-eye chili, chopped
- 600mls chicken stock
- 25g corn flour
- 60mls water
- 2 teaspoons fresh coriander

Directions:

1. Place the chicken, chickpeas (garbanzo beans), onion, carrot, chili, cumin, turmeric, cinnamon and stock (broth) into a large saucepan. Bring it to the boil, reduce the heat and simmer for 25 minutes. Add in the dates and apricots and simmer for 10 minutes. In a cup, mix the corn flour together with the water until it becomes a smooth paste. Pour the mixture into the saucepan and stir until it thickens. Add in the coriander (cilantro) and mix well. Serve with buckwheat or couscous.

Nutrition: Calories: 401 Net carbs: 3.6g Fat: 4.8g Fiber: 1.7g Protein: 29.2g

Prawn and Coconut Curry

Preparation time: 10 minutes

Cooking time: 5 minutes

Servings: 4

Ingredients:

- 400g tinned chopped tomatoes
- 400g large prawns (shrimps), shelled and raw
- 25g fresh coriander (cilantro) chopped
- 3 red onions, finely chopped
- 3 cloves of garlic, crushed
- 2 bird's eye chilies
- ½ teaspoon ground coriander (cilantro)
- ½ teaspoon turmeric
- 400mls (14fl Oz) coconut milk
- 1 teaspoons olive oil
- Juice of 1 lime

Directions:

1. Place the onions, garlic, tomatoes, chilies, lime juice, turmeric, ground coriander (cilantro), chilies and half of the fresh coriander (cilantro) into a blender and blitz until you have a smooth

curry paste. Heat the olive oil in a frying pan, add the paste and cook for 2 minutes. Stir in the coconut milk and warm it thoroughly. Add the prawns (shrimps) to the paste and cook them until they have turned pink and are completely cooked. Stir in the fresh coriander (cilantro). Serve with rice.

Nutrition: Calories: 322 Net carbs: 98.9g Fat: 11.8g Fiber: 8g Protein: 15.6g

Chicken and Bean Casserole

Preparation time: 15 minutes

Cooking time: 55 minutes

Servings: 4

Ingredients:

- 400g chopped tomatoes
- 400g tinned cannellini beans or haricot beans
- 8 chicken thighs, skin removed
- 2 carrots, peeled and finely chopped
- 2 red onions, chopped
- 4 sticks of celery
- 4 large mushrooms
- 2 red peppers (bell peppers), de-seeded and chopped
- 1 clove of garlic
- 2 teaspoons soy sauce
- 1 olive oil
- liters chicken stock (broth)

Directions:

1. Heat the olive oil in a saucepan, add the garlic and onions and cook for 5 minutes. Add in the

chicken and cook for 5 minutes then add the carrots, cannellini beans, celery, red peppers (bell peppers) and mushrooms. Pour in the stock (broth) soy sauce and tomatoes. Bring it to the boil, reduce the heat and simmer for 45 minutes. Serve with rice or new potatoes.

Nutrition: Calories: 509 Net carbs: 12.5g Fat: 6.5g Fiber: 1.1g Protein: 27.4g

Mussels in Red Wine Sauce

Preparation time: 5 minutes

Cooking time: 5 minutes

Servings: 2

Ingredients:

- 800g mussels
- 2 x 400g tins of chopped tomatoes
- 25g butter
- 1 fresh chives, chopped
- 1 fresh parsley, chopped
- 1 bird's-eye chili, finely chopped
- 4 cloves of garlic, crushed
- 400mls red wine
- Juice of 1 lemon

Directions:

1. Wash the mussels, remove their beards and set them aside. Heat the butter in a large saucepan and add in the red wine. Reduce the heat and add the parsley, chives, chili and garlic whilst stirring. Add in the tomatoes, lemon juice and mussels. Cover the saucepan and cook for 2-3.Remove the

saucepan from the heat and take out any mussels which haven't opened and discard them. Serve and eat immediately.

Nutrition: Calories: 364 Net carbs: 3.3g Fat: 4.9g Fiber: 0.7g Protein: 8.2g

Roast Balsamic Vegetables

Preparation time: 10 minutes

Cooking time: 45 minutes

Servings: 4

Ingredients:

- 4 tomatoes, chopped
- 2 red onions, chopped
- 3 sweet potatoes, peeled and chopped
- 100g red chicory (or if unavailable, use yellow)
- 100g kale, finely chopped
- 300g potatoes, peeled and chopped
- 5 stalks of celery, chopped
- 1 bird's-eye chili, de-seeded and finely chopped
- 2g fresh parsley, chopped
- 2gs fresh coriander (cilantro) chopped
- 3 teaspoons olive oil
- 2 teaspoons balsamic vinegar
- 1 teaspoon mustard
- Sea salt
- Freshly ground black pepper

Directions:

1. Place the olive oil, balsamic, mustard, parsley and coriander (cilantro) into a bowl and mix well. Toss all the remaining ingredients into the dressing and season with salt and pepper. Transfer the vegetables to an ovenproof dish and cook in the oven at 200C/400F for 45 minutes.

Nutrition: Calories: 310 Net carbs: 1.1g Fiber: 0.2g Protein: 0.2g

Tomato and Goat's Pizza

Preparation time: 15 minutes

Cooking time: 20 minutes

Servings: 2

Ingredients:

- 225g buckwheat flour
- 2 teaspoons dried yeast
- Pinch of salt
- 150mls slightly water
- 1 teaspoon olive oil
- For the Topping:
- 75g feta cheese, crumbled
- 75g peseta (or tomato paste)
- 1 tomato, sliced
- 1 red onion, finely chopped
- 25g rocket (arugula) leaves, chopped

Directions:

1. In a bowl, combine all the ingredients for the pizza dough then allow it to stand for at least an hour until it has doubled in size. Roll the dough out to a size to suit you. Spoon the passata onto

the base and add the rest of the toppings. Bake in the oven at 200C/400F for 15-20 minutes or until browned at the edges and crispy and serve.

Nutrition: Calories: 585 Net carbs: 77g Fat: 8.1g Fiber: 7.6g Protein: 22.9g

Tender Spiced Lamb

Preparation time: 20 minutes

Cooking time: 4 hours 20 minutes

Servings: 8

Ingredients:

- 1.35kg lamb shoulder
- 3 red onions, sliced
- 3 cloves of garlic, crushed
- 1 bird's eye chili, finely chopped
- 1 teaspoon turmeric
- 1 teaspoon ground cumin
- ½ teaspoon ground coriander (cilantro)
- ¼ teaspoon ground cinnamon
- 2 tablespoons olive oil

Directions:

1. In a bowl, combine the chili, garlic and spices with olive oil. Coat the lamb with the spice mixture and marinate it for an hour, or overnight if you can. Heat the remaining oil in a pan, add the lamb and brown it for 3-4 minutes on all sides to seal it. Place the lamb in an ovenproof dish. Add in the

red onions and cover the dish with foil. Transfer to the oven and roast at 170C/325F for 4 hours. The lamb should be extremely tender and falling off the bone. Serve with rice or couscous, salad or vegetables.

Nutrition: Calories: 455 Net carbs: 28g Fat: 9.8g Fiber: 11g Protein: 20g

Chili Cod Fillets

Preparation time: 10 minutes

Cooking time: 10 minutes

Servings: 4

Ingredients:

- 4 cod fillets each)
- 2 teaspoons fresh parsley, chopped
- 2 bird's-eye chilies (or more if you like it hot)
- 2 cloves of garlic, chopped
- 4 teaspoons olive oil

Directions:

1. Heat a of olive oil in a frying pan, add the fish and cook for 7-8 minutes or until thoroughly cooked, turning once halfway through. Remove and keep warm. Pour the remaining olive oil into the pan and add the chili, chopped garlic and parsley. Warm it thoroughly. Serve the fish onto plates and pour the warm chili oil over it.

Nutrition: Calories: 246 Net carbs: 5.5g Fat: 0.5g Fiber: 0.7g Protein: 18.5g

Steak and Mushroom Noodles

Preparation time: 10 minutes

Cooking time: 20 minutes

Servings: 4

Ingredients:

- 100g shitake mushrooms, halved, if large
- 100g chestnut mushrooms, sliced
- 150g udon noodles
- 75g kale, finely chopped
- 75g baby leaf spinach, chopped
- 2 sirloin steaks
- 2 teaspoons miso paste
- 2.5cm piece fresh ginger, finely chopped
- 2 teaspoons olive oil
- 1 star anise
- 1 red chili, finely sliced
- 1 red onion, finely chopped
- 1 fresh coriander (cilantro) chopped
- 1 liter (1½ pints) warm water

Directions:

1. Pour the water into a saucepan and add in the miso, star anise and ginger. Bring it to the boil, reduce the heat and simmer gently. In the meantime, cook the noodles according to their instructions then drain them. Heat the oil in a saucepan, add the steak and cook for around 2-3 minutes on each side (or 1-2 minutes, for rare meat).Remove the meat and set aside. Place the mushrooms, spinach, coriander (cilantro) and kale into the miso broth and cook for 5 minutes. In the meantime, heat the remaining oil in a separate pan and fry the chili and onion for 4 minutes, until softened. Serve the noodles into bowls and pour the soup on top. Thinly slice the steaks and add them to the top. Serve immediately.

Nutrition: Calories: 296 Net carbs: 24.6g Fat: 13.7g Fiber: 0.7g Protein: 32.9g

Masala Scallops

Preparation time: 10 minutes

Cooking time: 20 minutes

Servings: 4

Ingredients:

- 2 tablespoons olive oil
- 2 jalapenos, chopped
- 1 pound sea scallops
- A pinch of salt and black pepper
- ¼ teaspoon cinnamon powder
- 1 teaspoon garam masala
- 1 teaspoon coriander, ground
- 1 teaspoon cumin, ground
- 2 tablespoons cilantro, chopped

Directions:

1. Heat up a pan with the oil over medium heat, add the jalapenos, cinnamon and the other ingredients except the scallops and cook for 10 minutes.
2. Add the rest of the ingredients, toss, cook for 10 minutes more, divide into bowls and serve.

Nutrition: Calories: 251 Fat: 4g Fiber: 4g Carbs: 11g Protein: 17g

LUNCH

Oatless Ricotta Oatmeal

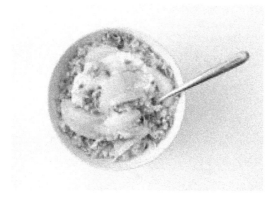

Preparation time: 5 minutes

Cooking time: 1 minute

Servings: 1

Ingredients:

- ½ cup organic ricotta cheese
- 4 tablespoons salted grass-fed butter
- ⅛ teaspoon ground cinnamon
- Sweetener to taste

Directions:

1. In a small microwave-safe bowl, mix the ricotta cheese, butter, cinnamon, and sweetener. Heat it in the microwave until hot, about 1 minute.

Nutrition: Calories: 578 Total fat: 56G Saturated fat: 35g Protein: 15G Cholesterol: 161MG Carbohydrates: 1G Fiber: 0G Net carbs: 1G Fat: 89% Carbs: 1% Protein: 10%

Lemon-Lavender Ricotta Pancakes

Preparation time: 5 minutes

Cooking time: 10 minutes

Servings: 2

Ingredients:

- 4 large free-range eggs
- ¼ cup organic ricotta cheese
- 2 teaspoons Sugar-Free Vanilla Bean Sweetener (here)
- 1 teaspoon freshly squeezed Meyer lemon juice
- 2 tablespoons coconut flour
- 1 tablespoon organic culinary lavender
- ½ teaspoon baking powder
- 1 tablespoon Golden Ghee (here)
- Grated zest of 1 Meyer lemon
- Grass-fed butter
- Sugar-free maple syrup

Directions:

1. In a blender, combine the eggs, ricotta cheese, sweetener, lemon juice, coconut flour, lavender, and baking powder. Blend on low for 10 seconds.

2. In a medium skillet, melt the ghee over medium heat. Pour about ¼ cup of the batter into the center of the pan. Cook the pancake until the bottom is brown and crispy, about 1 minute. Flip the pancake and cook the other side until brown and crispy, 30 seconds to 1 minute more. Repeat this step to cook 3 more pancakes.

Nutrition: Calories: 279 Total fat: 20G Saturated fat: 10G Protein: 18G Cholesterol: 398MG

Sweet Angel Eggs

Preparation time: 10 minutes

Cooking time: 15 Minutes

Servings: 2

Ingredients:

- 4 large free-range eggs, hardboiled and peeled
- 2 tablespoons mayonnaise
- 1 tablespoon Sugar-Free Vanilla Bean Sweetener (here; optional)
- ⅛ teaspoon ground cinnamon

Directions:

1. Halve the eggs lengthwise and scoop the yolks into a small bowl. Place the egg white halves on a plate.
2. Add the mayonnaise, sweetener (if using), and cinnamon to the yolks and mash them together.
3. Transfer the yolk mixture to a zipper-top plastic bag and cut off a small corner of the bag at the bottom. Pipe some of the yolk mixture into each egg white half. Serve.

Nutrition: Calories: 184 Total fat: 15G Saturated fat: 4G Protein: 12G Cholesterol: 331MG Carbohydrates: 1G Fiber: 0G Net carbs: 1G Fat: 72% Carbs: 2% Protein: 26%

Garlic and Thyme Baked Egg

Preparation time: 10 minutes

Cooking time: 5 minutes

Servings: 2

Butter and cream form the base of this delicious baked egg. Fragrant rosemary is a wonderful substitute for thyme if you prefer, but, in either case, use fresh herbs, not dried. This recipe takes only a few minutes to make, but you'll be thinking about it all day.

Ingredients:

- 1 garlic clove, minced
- Leaves from 1 thyme sprig
- 1½ teaspoons grated organic Parmesan cheese
- Pinch sea salt
- Freshly ground black pepper
- 1 tablespoon organic heavy (whipping) cream
- 1½ teaspoons Golden Ghee (here) or grass-fed butter
- 1 large free-range egg

Directions:

1. Preheat the oven to broil.

2. In a small bowl, mix the garlic, thyme, Parmesan cheese, salt, and a couple of cranks of pepper.

3. Combine the heavy cream and ghee in an 8-ounce ramekin. Place the ramekin on a rimmed baking sheet (for easier transport) and place it under the broiler until it begins to boil, about 1 minute (keep an eye on it as it could take less time).

4. Remove the baking sheet from the oven, and carefully and quickly crack the egg into the ramekin. Just as quickly spoon the herb mixture over the top of the egg. Place the baking sheet back under the broiler until the egg white is opaque, about 3 minutes more.

5. Remove the baked egg from the oven and let it rest and carryover cook for another minute. Serve immediately.

6. MAKE IT PALEO Increase the ghee to 1½ tablespoons and omit the Parmesan cheese and heavy cream. You'll still end up with a rich, buttery, herbed egg.

Nutrition: Calories: 182 Total fat: 17G Saturated fat: 9G Protein: 6G Cholesterol: 203MG Carbohydrates: 1G Fiber: 0G Net carbs: 1G Fat: 84% Carbs: 2% Protein: 14%

The Best Fried Eggs You'll Ever Eat

Preparation time: 5 minutes

Cooking time: 5 minutes

Servings: 1

Ingredients:

- 2 pinches onion powder
- Pinch ground cumin
- Pinch ground coriander
- Pinch sweet paprika
- Pinch chili powder
- Pinch dried parsley
- Pinch garlic salt
- Pinch sea salt

Directions:

1. 1½ teaspoons Golden Ghee (here)
2. 2 large free-range eggs
3. In a small bowl, combine the onion powder, cumin, coriander, paprika, chili powder, parsley, garlic salt, and sea salt. Set aside.
4. Over medium heat, melt the ghee in a small nonstick skillet.

5. Crack the eggs into the skillet and fry them until the whites are cooked, 3 to 5 minutes. Carefully flip them over (try not to break the yolks) and cook for 10 seconds more.
6. Transfer the eggs to a plate and sprinkle them with the spice mix (save any extra for later).

Nutrition: Calories: 205 Total fat: 17 Saturated fat: 7G Protein: 13G Cholesterol: 388MG Carbohydrates: 2G Fiber: 0G Net carbs: 2G Fat: 75% Carbs: 2% Protein: 23%

Shredded Chicken Bowl

Preparation Time: 10 minutes

Cooking time: 35 minutes

Total Time: 45 minutes

Serving 3-5

Ingredients:

- 1 jar of roasted tomato salsa or corn salsa/black bean
- 2-3 cups organic spinach (for your base)
- 1/2 cup cilantro
- Lime
- Coconut aminos
- 2 organic chicken breasts
- 1 jar of salsa Verde
- 2 ripe avocados
- 1/4-1/2 cup jalapeño sauerkraut

Directions:

1. Put/place the chicken breasts in a saucepan with one full salsa Verde jar and half a roasted tomato jar or black bean / corn salsa.

2. Cover and cook for 25 minutes on medium to low heat, or until chicken is cooked through.

3. When cooked through, remove the chicken and shred it with two forks, then put it back in the pot then heat for another 5 minutes-10 minutes.

4. Place your spinach base and drizzle with the coconut aminos in your serving bowls.

5. Add the shredded, cooked chicken into the bowl. (Vegetarian Sub Sweet Potatoes.) 6. For each bowl, add half a cut ripe avocado.

6. Add 2 spoonful of sauerkraut per bowl.

7. On each bowl, squeeze half a lime, and sprinkle with cilantro.

Nutrition: Calories 520 (2176 kJ) Cholesterol 85 mg 28% Sodium 1200 mg 50% Total Carbohydrate 54 g 18% Dietary Fiber 9 g

Buckwheat and Nut Loaf

Preparation time: 5 minutes

Cooking time: 10 minutes

Servings: 4

Ingredients:

- 2 tbsp. olive oil
- 225g/8oz mushrooms
- 2-3 carrots, finely diced
- 225g/8oz buckwheat
- 2-3 tbsp. fresh herbs, finely chopped eg: marjoram, oregano, thyme, parsley
- 225g/8oz nuts eg: almonds, hazelnuts, walnuts
- 2 eggs, beaten
- Salt and pepper

Directions:

1. Place the buckwheat in a pan with 350ml/1.5 cup pan of water and a pinch of salt. Take to boil. Cover and cook with the lid until all the water is absorbed-about 10-15 minutes.
2. Meanwhile, sauté the olive oil into the mushrooms and carrots until tender.

3. Blitz the food processor's nuts, until well chopped.
4. Stir in the eggs and combine the vegetables, cooked buckwheat, herbs and chopped nuts. If you are using tahini instead of eggs mix this with some water before stirring it into the buckwheat to create a thick pouring consistency.
5. Mix with pepper and salt.
6. Transfer to a oiled or lined loaf tin and bake for 30 minutes in the oven at gas mark 5/190C until set and just brown on top.

Nutrition: Calories 204.0 Total Fat 7.2 g Saturated Fat 0.9 g Cholesterol 67.7 mg Dietary Fiber 0.9 g Sugars 2.6 g Protein

DINNER

Zucchini Carpaccio with Natural Mackerel

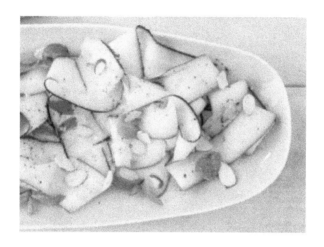

Preparation time: 5 minutes

Cooking time: 15 minutes

Servings: 12

Ingredients:

- 240 g of mackerel fillets
- 400g of Courgettes
- 80 ml of extra virgin olive oil
- The juice of one lemon
- Parsley
- A few mint leaves
- Some grain of pink pepper
- Salt

Directions:

1. Cut the Zucchini into thin slices, put them in a tray and add the salt. Leave the Courgettes to rest for 10 minutes, in this way they will take out all the liquids contained and become softer.
2. We prepare the dressing - In a bowl we put the extra virgin olive oil and the juice of a lemon, add the salt and begin to mix quickly with a whisk to create an emulsion.

3. We combine the finely chopped parsley and some crushed pink pepper, we mix again until everything is mixed.

4. We prepare the zucchini Carpaccio - take the slices of zucchini, dry them with kitchen paper and place them in a bowl. Pour over the dressing and mix until everything is mixed.

5. We serve in a single serving dish, arranging the Carpaccio as a base and on top we have the Grilled Mackerel Fillets adding a drizzle of oil.

Nutrition: Calories: 216 Fat: 16.9g Protein: 13.3g Carbohydrate: 3.4g Fiber: 0.9g

Couscous with Vegetables Au Gratin

Preparation time: 5 minutes

Cooking time: 15 minutes

Servings: 12

Ingredients:

- 150g of couscous
- 250ml of hot water
- Half a red pepper
- Half a yellow pepper
- A medium courgette
- Two medium potatoes
- Parsley to taste
- Extra virgin olive oil to taste
- Salt and pepper
- 20-30g of parmesan already grated

Directions:

1. Cut the peppers and courgette into small cubes. Steam the vegetables for 5-10 minutes depending on the quantity, taste before removing from the steamer.

2. Take the hot water and pour it over the couscous taking into consideration the instructions of the brand you have chosen. Cover the bowl containing the couscous and leave it for 10-15 minutes, until the water has been completely absorbed.
3. Take the ready-made couscous and shell it with a fork, add the vegetables, salt and pepper, chopped parsley and a drizzle of oil.
4. Take the potatoes and cut them finely with the mandolin, lay them half on the bottom of an oiled oven pan, fill with the couscous, spread another row of chopped potatoes like chips, a drizzle of oil and finally the parmesan. Bake at 200 ° until the surface is golden brown and then for about 20-25 minutes.

Nutrition: Calories: 219 Fat: 16.9g Protein: 13.3g Carbohydrate: 3.4g Fiber: 0.9g

Steamed Spelled With Salmon and Tomatoes

Preparation time: 5 minutes

Cooking time: 15 minutes

Servings: 12

Ingredients:

- 200g spelled
- 3 long salad tomatoes
- 100g of Fjord salmon
- A small fennel
- A little chopped parsley
- A drizzle of extra virgin olive oil
- Salt and pepper

Directions:

1. Soak the spelled for 12 hours, and read the directions on the package here because times vary depending on the brand. Steam the spelled with the steamer in very small holes or with a colander to be placed on a pan, perhaps the one for the pasta without letting the colander touch the water. Here too times vary according to the

brand of spelled used, they are longer than normal cooking and sometimes they can double. You must use two parts of water and one of cereal to regulate cooking. The advantage in this case is that the spelled will have a better flavor and texture.

2. When the spelled is cooked, chop the salmon and add it to the steamer, leave it for 2-3 minutes maximum with the lid closed, or you can add the salmon cold.

3. Take the spelled with salmon, put it in a bowl and add two three diced salad tomatoes, add a drizzle of oil, a little chopped parsley, the cubed fennel and season with salt and pepper.

Nutrition: Calories: 345 Fat: 21.9g Protein: 13.3g Carbohydrate: 3.4g Fiber: 0.9g

SNACKS & DESSERTS

Kale and Apple Cake

Preparation time: 15 minutes

Cooking time: 40 minutes

Servings: 4

Ingredients:

- 3 cups inexactly pressed, (200g) kale crude, woody stalks disposed of)

- 3 eggs

- 1/2 cup vegetable oil

- 2 teaspoons vanilla concentrate

- 1/2 cup fruit purée

- 3/4 cup granulated sugar

- 2 apples stripped and ground

- 2 cups plain flour

- 2 teaspoons heating powder

- ½ teaspoon salt

Directions:

1. Preheat grill to 180C/350F. Oil and line 2 x 8" (20cm) round cake tins with heating paper. Tear the kale leaves into reduced pieces and bubble or steam for a couple of moments until delicate.

2. Revive by running under virus water, channel, and puree well with a hand blender. It will even now be marginally stringy. Put in a safe spot.

3. Beat the eggs, oil, vanilla, fruit purée, and sugar together well with an electric blender. Beat in the kale puree and ground apple.

4. Filter in the flour, heating powder, and salt and tenderly consolidate, considering not to overmix at this stage.

5. Fill the readied tins and bake within 30 minutes. Cool within 2 minutes in the tins, and afterward, turn onto a wire rack to cool totally.

Nutrition: Calories: 200 Carbs: 23g Fat: 11g Protein: 4g

Low Carb Blender Sherbet

Preparation time: 15 minutes

Cooking time: 0 minutes

Servings: 2

Ingredients:

- 1 (3 ounces) box without sugar gelatin (any flavor)

- 1 tbsp substantial whipping cream

- 1/3 cup bubbling water

- 1/3 cup super-cold water

- about 1.5 cups ice

Directions:

1. Empty the dry gelatin into a medium-size bowl. Include 1/3 cup bubbling water and mix until the gelatin is very much broken down.

2. Include 1/3 cup of freezing water and 1 tbsp of substantial whipping cream, and mix. Spot 1.5 cups of ice into a decent quality blender and pour

the gelatin blend over the ice. Mix until smooth and serve right away.

Nutrition: Calories: 60 Carbs: 0g Fat: 6g Protein: 1g

Pistachio Fluff Salad

Preparation time: 15 minutes

Cooking time: 0 minutes

Servings: 3

Ingredients:

- 2 boxes JELL-O Instant Pistachio pudding blend

- 1 can squashed pineapple

- 16 oz Cool Whip, defrosted

- 1 sack smaller than usual marshmallows

- maraschino fruits, for embellish

Directions:

1. In an enormous bowl, join pudding blend in with squashed pineapple. Blend in with a wooden spoon until the pudding blend is mixed with pineapple fluids.

2. Include Cool Whip and smaller than regular marshmallows. Cover and refrigerate for 4 hours, or medium-term.

3. Present with maraschino fruits as an embellishment. Or then again, whenever wanted, add fruits to lighten directly before serving.

Nutrition: Calories: 145 Carbs: 10g Fat: 3g Protein: 0g

Watergate Salad

Preparation time: 15 minutes

Cooking time: 0 minutes

Servings: 2

Ingredients:

- 2 jars squashed pineapple in juice, undrained

- 1 bundle pistachio moment pudding

- 1 tub solidified whipped beating, defrosted

- 1 cup smaller than usual marshmallows

- 1/2 cup toasted walnuts, hacked

Directions:

1. In a medium bowl, mix the pineapple jars' full substance and the pudding blend until smooth. Overlay in whipped fixing and marshmallows. Cover and refrigerate in any event for 60 minutes. Sprinkle walnuts on top before serving.

Nutrition: Calories: 190 Carbs: 22g Fat: 11g Protein: 1g

Strawberry Pretzel Salad

Preparation time: 15 minutes

Cooking time: 10 minutes

Servings: 4

Ingredients:

Pretzel Crust:

- 3 1/2 cups pretzels, squashed

- 1/4 cup sugar

- 1/2 cup unsalted spread, dissolved

Cream Cheese Filling:

- 8 oz cream cheddar, mellowed

- 1/2 cup sugar

- 8 oz cool whip or whipped cream (solidly whipped)

Strawberry Jell-O Topping:

- 1 lb. new strawberries, hulled and cut

- 2 cups bubbling water

- 6 oz strawberry jello powder

Directions:

1. Preheat stove to 350°F. Put aside a 9x13 inch glass preparing dish. Spot pretzels in a Ziplock sack, seal and pound with a moving pin to smash daintily.

2. In a medium bowl, mix the liquefied margarine and sugar. Include the squashed pretzels and blend to cover. Press the pretzel blend into the preparing dish, and afterward heat for 10 minutes. Expel from broiler.

3. In a medium bowl, consolidate jello powder with bubbling water. Mix gradually for one moment until broke down and put in a safe spot.

4. In a large bowl, beat the cream cheddar and sugar until soft. Utilizing a huge spatula, crease in the cool whip until equitably mixed.

5. When the prepared pretzels are cool, spread the cream cheddar, equitably on top until level over the dish. At that point, chill for at any rate 30 minutes.

6. While chilling, you can wash, body, and cut the strawberries. Tenderly spot the cut strawberries onto the filling in a solitary layer. Include any residual strawberries top as a fractional second layer.

7. When the jello blend is room temperature, spill over the strawberries utilizing a spoon's rear for even dispersion. Chill for, in any event, two hours. Serve and appreciate!

Nutrition: Calories: 159 Carbs: 23g Fat: 6g Protein: 4g

Sheet Pan Apple Pie Bake

Preparation time: 15 minutes

Cooking time: 30 minutes

Servings: 4

Ingredients:

- 8 flour tortillas, 8 inches

- 4 tbsp unsalted spread

- 8 Granny Smith apples, stripped, cored, and cleaved

- 3/4 cup sugar, partitioned

- 3 tsp cinnamon, partitioned

- 1 tbsp lemon juice, pressed

- Serving thoughts - discretionary

- whipped cream

- frozen yogurt

- caramel sauce

Directions:

1. Preheat stove to 400°F. Put aside a medium preparing sheet.

2. On a medium preparing sheet, orchestrate 6 tortillas in a blossom petal design with a few creeps outside the dish and a few crawls of cover.

3. Put the 7th tortilla in the center. Put an enormous skillet on medium-high warmth. Include spread, slashed apples, 1/2 cup sugar, and 2 tsp cinnamon. Sauté the apples for 8-10 minutes until they begin to relax, mixing naturally with a wooden spoon.

4. Spoon apple blend from skillet over tortillas on prepared sheet. Spread out to make an even layer. Overlay the folds of the tortilla outside the dish over the apples.

5. Spot the eighth tortilla in the center to cover the hole. Blend staying 1/4 cup sugar with 1 tsp cinnamon. Sprinkle equally over the tortillas.

6. Spot another preparing dish on top to hold the tortillas set up and heat for 20 minutes. Expel from the stove and permit to cool for 5-10 minutes. Present with discretionary frozen

yogurt, whipped cream, and caramel sauce. Appreciate!

Nutrition: Calories: 340 Carbs: 49g Fat: 16g Protein: 2g

Heaven on Earth Cake

Preparation time: 15 minutes

Cooking time: 10 minutes

Servings: 4

Ingredients:

- 1 box Angel nourishment cake or 1 arranged Angel Food Cake

- 1 bundle (3.4 ounces) moment vanilla pudding

- 1/2 cups milk

- 1 cup harsh cream

- 1 can (21 ounces) cherry pie filling

- 1 tub (8 ounces) Cool Whip

- 1 tablespoon almond bits, toasted

Directions:

1. Heat fluffy cake as indicated by bundle's bearings. Permit to cool and cut into 3D shapes.

2. In a bowl, consolidate pudding blend, milk, and acrid cream and beat until smooth. Put in a safe

spot. In a 9x13 preparing dish, organize 1/2 of cake solid shapes layer.

3. Spoon 2/3 of cherry over cake. Spot the staying 1/2 of the cake over pie filling. Spoon pudding over cake and spread equally. Spoon and spread whipped besting over pudding layer.

4. Decorate the cake with the rest of the pie filling and toasted almonds. Chill for around 4 to 5 hours.

Nutrition: Calories: 417 Carbs: 66g Fat: 10g Protein: 9g

Strawberry Upside-Down Cake

Preparation time: 15 minutes

Cooking time: 50 minutes

Servings: 4

Ingredients:

- 2 cup new strawberries squashed

- 2 3-oz strawberry Jell-O

- 3 cup little marshmallows

- 18 & 1/4 oz. strawberry cake blend + fixings to get ready cake blend

- Cool Whip

Directions:

1. Take your two cups of strawberries and pound them with a fork. Fill a lubed 9x13 in a cake container. Sprinkle strawberry Jell-O over the highest point of the strawberries.

2. At that point, sprinkle the marshmallows over the Jell-O. Plan cake blend, as indicated by bundle headings. Pour over the marshmallows.

3. Heat at 350 degrees for 40-50 minutes or until cake tests are done. Let sit for around 15 minutes and afterward, run a blade around the outside of the cake. Flip onto a serving plate. Refrigerate. Present with Cool Whip. Store scraps in the fridge.

Nutrition: Calories: 189 Carbs: 39g Fat: 5g Protein: 4g

SIDES

Nutty Green Beans

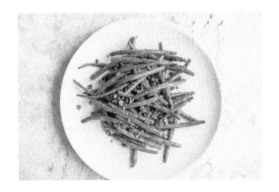

Preparation time: 10 minutes

Cooking time: 5 minutes

Servings: 2

Ingredients:

- 2 tbsp. each chunky-style peanut butter

- 2 tbsp sherry

- 2 tsp. oyster sauce

- 1 garlic clove, minced

- 1/2 tsp. minced pared ginger root

- 2 cups cooked frozen French-style green beans (hot)

Directions:

1. In a small saucepan, combine peanut butter, sherry, oyster sauce, garlic, and ginger; bring to a boil. Reduce heat and let simmer, continually stirring until the mixture is creamy, about 1 minute. Pour peanut butter mixture over hot green beans and serve immediately.

Nutrition: Calories 157 Fat 8 g Carbs 3 g Protein 7 g

Vegetable-Cottage Cheese

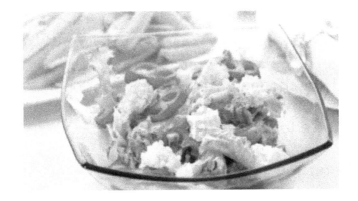

Preparation time: 10 minutes

Cooking time: 0 minutes

Servings: 1

Ingredients:

- 6 cherry tomatoes
- ½ cup cottage cheese
- 2 tbsp. chopped scallion (green onion)
- 2 pimiento-stuffed green olives, sliced
- 1 tbsp. chopped fresh parsley (optional)
- Lettuce leaves

Directions:

1. Cut five tomatoes into quarters; reserve remaining tomato for garnish. Mix all the fixing except lettuce in a small bowl and garnish; mix well. Line a salad plate with lettuce leaves, top with cheese mixture, and garnish with a reserved cherry tomato.

Nutrition: Calories 187 Fat 8 g Carbs 9 g Protein 20 g

Grilled Asparagus with Caper Vinaigrette

Preparation time: 10 minutes

Cooking time: 5 minutes

Servings: 6

Ingredients:

- 1 ½ lb. asparagus spears, trimmed

- 2 tsp. caper, coarsely chopped

- 1 tbsp. red wine vinegar

- 1 garlic clove, minced

- 3 tbsp. Extra virgin olive oil

- ¼ cup small basil leaves

- ½ tsp. Dijon mustard

- Cooking spray

- ½ tsp. Kosher salt, divided

- ¼ tsp. ground black pepper

Directions:

1. Preheat grill to medium-high heat. Place asparagus in a shallow dish. Add 1 tbsp oil and ¼ tsp, and salt, tossing well to coat. Place asparagus on grill rack coated with cooking spray.

2. Grill 4 minutes or until crisp-tender, turning after 2 minutes. Combine remaining ¼ tsp: salt, vinegar, mustard, and garlic.

3. Stir with a whisk. Slowly pour the remaining 2 tbsp of oil into the vinegar mixture, continually stirring with a whisk. Stir in capers. Arrange asparagus on a serving platter. Drizzle with vinaigrette and sprinkle with basil.

Nutrition: Calories 89 Fat 6.9g Carbs 4.7g Protein 2.8g

Cheesy Asparagus

Preparation time: 10 minutes

Cooking time: 15 minutes

Servings: 4

Ingredients:

- 1 lb. asparagus, trimmed

- 2 tbsp. olive oil

- ½ cup Parmesan cheese, shredded

- ½ cup mozzarella cheese, shredded

- 1 tbsp. Italian seasoning

- Black pepper and sea salt to taste:

Directions:

1. Warm oven to 400° F. Line a baking sheet with foil or parchment paper. Mix the asparagus with olive oil, sea salt, black pepper, plus half of the Italian seasoning.

2. Put in a single layer on the lined baking sheet. Roast in the oven for about 8 minutes, until the

asparagus is bright green and just starting to soften.

3. Mix the mozzarella plus Parmesan cheese, then sprinkle over the asparagus. Top with remaining Italian seasoning. Return to the oven within 7 minutes, until the cheese is melted and golden.

Nutrition: Calories 160 Fat 12g Carbs 3g Protein 8g

Stuffed Avocado

Preparation time: 10 minutes

Cooking time: 0 minutes

Servings: 2

Ingredients:

- 2 tbsp. light mayonnaise

- 1 tsp. chopped fresh chives

- ¼ cup peeled and diced cucumber

- 2 tsp. sriracha, plus more for drizzling

- 1 small avocado (pitted and peeled)

- ½ tsp. furikake

- 2 tsp. gluten-free soy sauce

Directions:

1. Mix mayonnaise, sriracha, and chives in a medium bowl. Add cucumber, plus chive, and gently toss. Cut the avocado open, remove the pit and peel the skin or spoon the avocado out.

Fill the avocado halves equally with crab salad. Top with furikake and drizzle with soy sauce.

Nutrition: Calories 194 Fat 13g Carbs 7g Protein 12g

Kale Sauté

Preparation time: 10 minutes

Cooking time: 15 minutes

Servings: 2

Ingredients:

- 1 chopped red onion

- 3 tbsps. coconut aminos

- 2 tbsps. olive oil

- 1 lb. torn kale

- 1 tbsp. chopped cilantro

- 1 tbsp. lime juice

- 2 minced garlic cloves

Directions:

1. Heat-up a pan with the olive oil over medium heat, add the onion and the garlic, and sauté for 5 minutes. Add the kale and the other ingredients, toss, cook over medium heat for 10 minutes, divide between plates and serve.

Nutrition: Calories 200 Fat 7.1 g Carbs 6.4 g Protein 6 g

Garlic Hummus

Preparation time: 5 minutes

Cooking time: 10 minutes

Servings: 4

Ingredients:

- 3 tbsp freshly squeezed lemon juice

- all-purpose salt-free seasoning

- 3 tbsps. sesame tahini

- 4 garlic cloves

- 15 oz. no-salt-added garbanzo beans, rinsed & drained

- 2 tbsps. olive oil

Directions:

1. Place all the fixing in a food processor, then pulse until smooth. Serve immediately.

Nutrition: Calories 103 Fat 5 g Carbs 11 g Protein 4 g

Sage Carrots

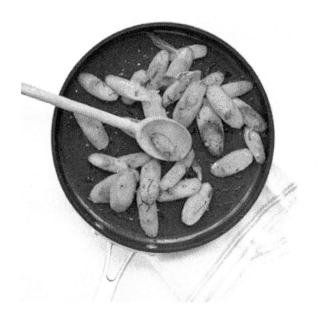

Preparation Time: 10 minutes

Cooking Time: 30 minutes

Servings: 2

Ingredients:

- 2 tsp sweet paprika

- 1 tbsp chopped sage

- 2 tbsp olive oil

- 1 lb. peeled and roughly cubed carrots

- ¼ tsp black pepper

- 1 chopped red onion

Directions:

1. In a baking pan, combine the carrots with the oil and the other ingredients, toss and bake at 380 0F for 30 minutes. Divide between plates and serve.

Nutrition: Calories: 200 Fat: 8.7 g Carbs: 7.9 g Protein: 4 g

Carrot, Tomato, And Arugula Quinoa Pilaf

Preparation Time: 10 minutes

Cooking Time: 22 minutes

Servings: 4

Ingredients:

- 2 teaspoons extra virgin olive oil

- ½ red onion, chopped

- 1 cup quinoa, raw

- 2 cups vegetable or chicken broth

- 1 tsp fresh lovage, chopped

- 1 carrot, chopped

- 1 tomato, chopped

- 1 cup baby arugula

Directions:

1. Heat-up olive oil in a saucepan over medium heat and add the red onion. Cook and stir until translucent, about 5 minutes.

2. Lower the heat, stir in quinoa, and toast, continually stirring, for 2 minutes. Stir in the broth, black pepper, and thyme.

3. Raise the heat to be high and bring it to a boil. Cover, adjust to low and simmer for 5 minutes. Stir in the carrots, cover, and simmer until all water is absorbed about 10 more minutes.

4. Turn off the heat, add tomatoes, arugula and lovage and let sit for 5 minutes. Add salt and pepper to taste.

Nutrition: Calories: 165 Fat: 4g Carbs: 27g Protein: 6g

Bake Kale Walnut

Preparation Time: 10 minutes

Cooking Time: 30 minutes

Servings: 4

Ingredients:

- 1 medium red onion, finely chopped
- ¼ cup extra virgin olive oil
- 2 cups baby kale
- ½ cup half-and-half cream
- ½ cup walnuts, coarsely chopped
- 1/3 cup dry breadcrumbs
- ½ tsp ground nutmeg
- Salt and pepper to taste
- ¼ cup dry breadcrumbs
- 2 tbsp. extra virgin olive oil

Directions:

1. Warm oven to 350 degrees F. In a skillet, sauté onion in olive oil until tender. In a large bowl, combine cooked onion, kale, cream, walnuts, breadcrumbs, nutmeg, salt, and pepper to taste, mixing well.

2. Transfer to a greased 1-1/2-qt—baking dish. Combine topping ingredients and sprinkle over the kale mixture. Bake, uncovered, within 30 minutes or until lightly browned.

Nutrition: Calories: 555 Fat: 31g Carbs: 65g Protein: 26g

Arugula with Apples and Pine Nuts

Preparation Time: 10 minutes

Cooking Time: 8 minutes

Servings: 4

Ingredients:

- 2 tbsp extra virgin olive oil

- 2 cloves garlic, slivered

- 2 tbsp pine nuts

- 1 apple, peeled, cored, and chopped

- 10 oz. arugula

- Salt and pepper to taste

Directions:

1. Warm-up olive oil in a large skillet or wok over low heat. Put the garlic, pine nuts, and apple. Cook within 3 to 5 minutes.

2. Adjust the heat to medium and add the arugula. Stir and cook another 2 to 3 minutes—season with salt and pepper to taste.

Nutrition: Calories: 121 Fat: 9g Carbs: 8g Protein: 3g

Kale Green Bean Casserole

Preparation Time: 5 minutes

Cooking Time: 40 minutes

Servings: 4

Ingredients:

- 1 ½ cups milk

- 1 cup sour cream

- 1 cup mushrooms, chopped

- 2 cups green beans, chopped

- 2 cups kale, chopped

- ¼ cup capers, drained

- ¼ cup walnuts, crushed

Directions:

1. Warm oven to 375 degrees F and lightly greases a casserole dish. Whisk the milk and sour cream together in a large bowl.

2. Add mushrooms, green beans, kale, and capers. Pour into the casserole dish and top with the

crushed walnuts. Bake uncovered in the preheated oven until bubbly and browned on top, about 40 minutes.

Nutrition: Calories: 130 Fat: 6g Carbs: 14g Protein: 2g